Mas-tur-ba-tion

by Marilyn Coffey

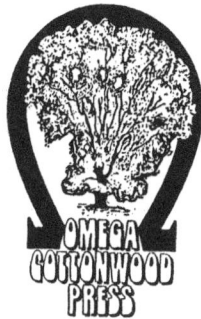

OMEGA
COTTONWOOD
PRESS

Omaha, NE

Paperback ISBN-13: 978-0-9626317-9-5
Cataloging in Publication Data on file with publisher.

Omega Cottonwood Press
13518 L St.
Omaha, NE 68137

Printed in the United States
10 9 8 7 6 5 4 3 2 1

Table of Contents

Is Masturbation a Sin?

"The subject of masturbation
is quite inexhaustible."

--Sigmund Freud

Is masturbation a sin?

If it is, nobody's saying so -- at least not to this reporter.

Obviously, this question is literally a religious one; only religious leaders speak in terms of "sin," which, by Random House dictionary definition, is a "transgression of a <u>divine</u> law" (emphasis mine). In a broader sense, of course, sin is simply a transgression of any religious or moral principle, or any <u>serious</u> offense or fault (again, emphasis mine).

Still, the authority that most people would, it seemed to me, turn to in such

a matter would be their church. There-
fore, to answer the question, I asked
fifteen religious leaders from a wide
variety of faiths, to address this issue.
I asked Baha'i, Buddhist, several kinds
of Christian (Evangelical Free, Presbyte-
rian, Roman Catholic), Jewish, Hindu,
Muslim, Native American, Pagan, Sikh,
Sufi and Unitarian-Universalist leaders.
Not one would speak.

But, since "silence on sex, in sharp
contrast to relatively free talk on other
topics, is the most effective device for
communicating guilt and anxiety and
apathy and ambivalent fascination and
revulsion," according to Dr. Robert A.
Harper in his *Sex and American Attitudes*, I decided not to fall silent on this
question, but rather explore it myself,
as best I could without any assistance
from the clergy.

The Bible, that great reference work on
questions of sin, does not mention
masturbation by name. It may allude to
the subject three times, once each in
Genesis, Ezekiel, and First Corinthians.

The Genesis reference (38:8-10) contains the famous Onan quote -- that thou shall not "spill your seed." Some critics say this means you must not masturbate; others say that the Onan offense is coitus interruptus, not masturbation. In any case, the matter doesn't clarify the question of whether or not masturbation (including female masturbation, with no "seed" to spill) is a sin.

In the Ezekiel quote (16:17), God accuses Jerusalem of having committed "whoredom" with graven images of men, which some interpret as a reference to dildoes, but it's not clear whether God's upset with the whoredom per se, or the choice of human figures as dildoes.

In the 1 Corinthians quote (6:9- 10), Paul, writing to the Corinthians, says that the "unrighteous shall not inherit the kingdom of God." Among the "unrighteous" are "abusers of themselves," presumably masturbators if the translators of the King James version (finished in 1611) used the term as it is used today. In my home county, at least, "self abuse" is a euphemism for "masturbation" (just as "passed away" is a euphemism for "died.") Other euphemisms for masturbation are "a different kind of pleasure," "amusing oneself" and "jollification."

Except for Paul's ambiguous listing, the Bible, per se, says nothing directly about masturbation. The guilt that surrounds this sexual act seems to be caused by severely disapproving attitude of authority figures, namely, the clergy.

When ancient Jews and Christians banned masturbation, they were ignorant of its harmlessness. Also, in those earlier cultures, girls married at 13 or 14, boys at 15 or 16. They did not have to wait, to delay sexual gratification for years, as is the norm in our society.

In the case of the Roman Catholic church, the disapproval of male masturbation is clear. The Catholic church condemns the practice of male masturbation as a mortal sin, according to Urban T. Holmes III in his *The Sexual Person: The Church's Role in Human Sexual Development*, written in 1970.

This despite the fact that 92 per cent of adolescent boys masturbate. Masturbation, say the medical doctors, is a universal phenomenon, practiced in all classes of society and in all types of culture. Indeed, according to recent scientific studies, fetuses masturbate in the womb.

Masturbation is not a learned response; it is an inborn instinct.

Most American men (and a solid majority of women) have masturbated at some time.

At the other end of the church spectrum from the Roman Catholics, the Unitarian Church, in 1971, sponsored a series of sex education films for young people. The films included pictures of both men and women masturbating.

So church attitudes toward masturbation certainly don't seem universal.

Where did masturbation get such a bad name anyway?

At the beginning of the 18th century, a pamphlet in England and a dissertation in France stirred up readers. The crusade, led by physicians, appealed to a sense of shame. One of the most vocal doctors, Dr. Kellogg, specialized in "curing" masturbation, so of course it was in his best interest to establish that masturbating was a disease. He and others wrote violent books claiming that masturbation caused impotence, epilepsy, consumption, blindness, imbecility, insanity and death.

Prior to this time, masturbation was rarely mentioned. This early crusade may have been the first time science ever scrutinized the subject.

Perhaps this was when masturbation was said to mean "to defile with the hand." Actually, the term comes down to us from Latin, its original meaning obscured by time, according to the *Oxford English Dictionary*.

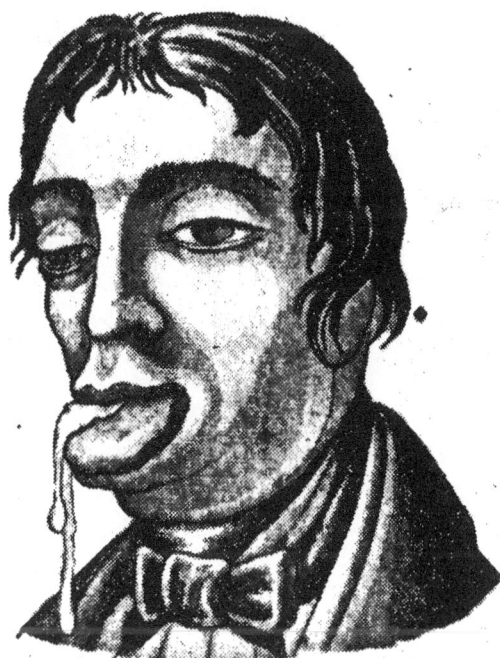

The meagre appearance of the feature through Onanism.

This 1853 scare-drawing shows the disastrous results predicted for males who masturbated.

Even as late as 1900, masturbation was considered a disease -- or at least a disorder -- by medical doctors. Here's what F. R. Sturgis, MD, recommends in his book, *How to Treat Masturbation*:

● administer a mild tonic

● prescribe cold baths

● suggest out-of-door exercises (but NOT horseback riding, biking, climbing poles, etc.)

● hypnotize the masturbator and tell him or her to stop.

● restrain the body at night

● install a close-meshed wire cage from the waist to the thighs, a cage that is bowed out around the genitals. Padlock it shut BEFORE bed. Put nightclothes on OVER the cage

● whip the masturbator

● blister the genitals

● castrate the masturbator (if male) or cauterize or amputate the clitoris (if female)

Dr. Albert Ellis writes that our anti-masturbation attitudes stem from our puritan background, marked by a tendency to feel guilty when unqualifiedly enjoying ourselves. Human beings, he feels, punish themselves senselessly by depriving themselves of masturbation.
"It is certainly better for youngsters and oldsters to copulate and to pet, when they wish to do so, than merely to masturbate. But if the choice is between autoeroticism and abstinence, who in his right mind would pick the latter?" writes Dr. Ellis.

In other cultures, attitudes toward masturbation are more tolerant and permissive, according to the American Medical Association. Parents in other cultures don't disapprove of infant masturbation, for instance. Some cultures have a special word for masturbation by women. Some carve images of masturbators on the facades of their temples. And in many places (among the Basutos and Kaffirs, the Hottentots of Africa), masturbation is treated as a very ordinary fact of life, cropping up repeatedly in stories and legends.

Today, the scientific community has changed its attitude toward masturbation dramatically. Today, masturbation is considered an integral part of human sexuality.

The attitude of modern psychologists is markedly different than the disapproving stance of the Catholic church. "Actually, medical science tells us that masturbation ... is one of the quite normal experiences of growing up," writes Mary Steichen Calderone, M.D., in her *Release from Sexual Tensions*.

This, despite the fact that some people still believe masturbation is a serious sin, a major sign of immorality. These people would stop masturbation by force, if necessary. These attitudes are based on the attitudes of Christian religion, says N. Lukianowicz, MD. Such negativity often causes neurotic reactions in people. Masturbation, says

John D. LaTendresse, MD, does not cause neurotic problems. Disturbed people sometimes use masturbation to interfere with social life, prevent hetero-sexual involvement, etc.

Fortunately, this negative attitude is disappearing. In the scientific community, masturbation is generally considered not simply "normal & natural, but even necessary & healthy," according to Eda J. LeShan in her *Sex & Your Teenager: A Guide for Parents*. Helpful sexologists such as Dr. Ruth aid in this change.

Sex educators recommend masturbation to release sexual tension and to learn about your own orgasmic pattern.

Masturbation lays the groundwork for a full adult sexual relationship, writes Dr. Calderone. Kinsey maintained that the experience gained by a masturbating woman helps her orgasm in intercourse.

Of course, a woman may prefer orgasm by her own hand, since that's generally considered stronger than orgasm in intercourse.

It's difficult, say the experts, to practice self-stimulation to excess. Why? After awhile, a person loses desire and quite naturally stops for a time.

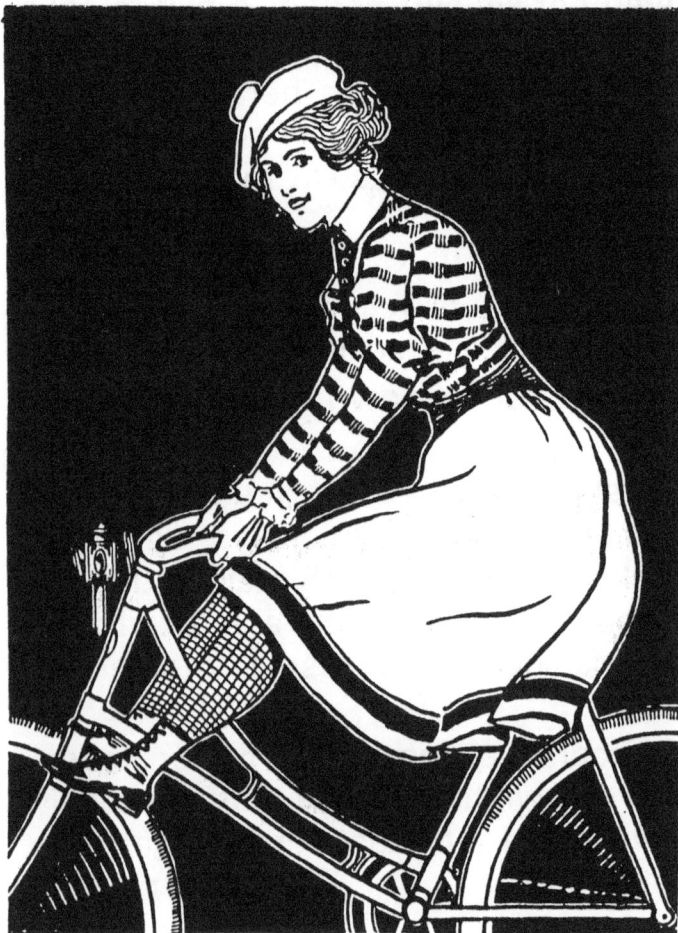

Arguments for Masturbation

It is easily available.

It doesn't interfer with the sex rights of others.

It is free from venereal infection.

It is free from pregnancy or abortion.

It helps develop erotic fantasy (useful later in heterosexual coupling).

It calms sexual urges and emotions.

It provides excitement in our "quick relief" culture.

It can be practiced when other forms of gratification aren't available.

It can be interspersed with non-sexual occupations (such as sewing).

It needs no preliminary steps.

It needs no special apparatus.

It needs no hygenic precautions.

It can be practiced when one is sick
and lying in bed.

It can be practiced when dual sex
isn't available (as in prison, armed
forces, sailors, students in one-sex
schools, etc.).

It is obviously harmless and even
beneficial.

-- adapted from Albert Ellis, Ph.D.

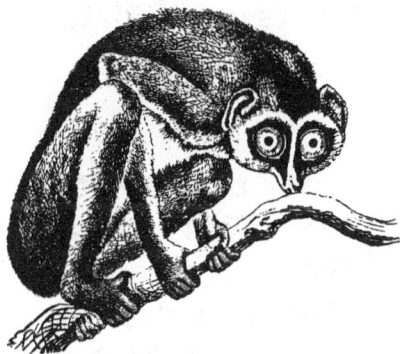

Who, besides Man, Masturbates?

In our patriarchal society, masturbation is treated -- by most writers -- as an activity indulged in only by human men. Yet many other animals stimulate their sexual organs: primates, elephants, dogs, cats, horses, bulls, goats, ferrets, sheep, camels, bears, hyenas, parrots, and women, to name a few.

Some primates evidently masturbate to orgasm, using their hand (the monkey's favorite), foot, mouth, tail or rubbing against the ground or some other object. Male elephants masturbate with their trunk or compress their penis between their hindlegs (to their jollification!) Dogs and cats masturbate by licking themselves.

Male horses flop their penises to ejaculate, mares rub themselves against objects (and ponies, those romantics, close their eyes while masturbating!) Bulls and goats use their forelegs as a stimulus, and goats, the envy of many a human male, are into autofellatio (or sucking themselves off). A ferret bitch was seen masturbating on a pebble.

Stags rub trees until they ejaculate. Sheep and camels press against any

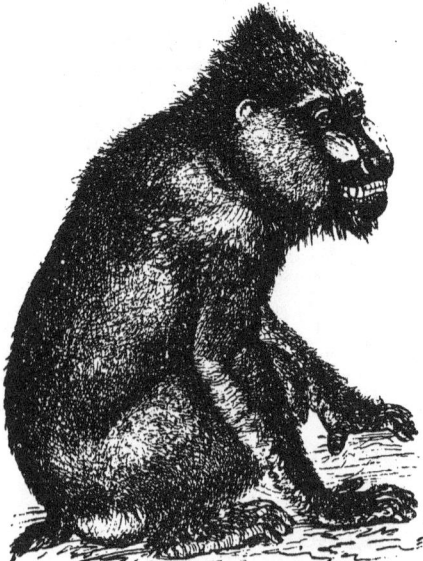

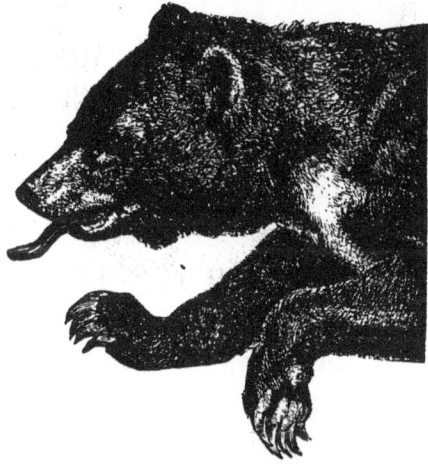

convenient object. And hyenas specialize in mutual masturbation (69).

Needless to say, female human masturbators also abound. A majority of women in our culture masturbate, say sex experts. How do they do it? There are three commonly favored forms: vaginal, clitoral or ureteral.

Vaginal masturbators like dildoes (artificial penises) of all kinds -- made of clay, wax, glass, wood, cork, ivory, leather, hardened rubber, plastic, ebony or paper. Among female favorites are vibrators, candles, pencils, crochet hooks, corks, tumblers, toothbrushes, -- and of course, different fruits and vegetables. The banana (peeled) is very popular as is the peeled cucumber. Or a jet of hot water. Root vegetables are enjoyed, too -- the turnip and the carrot. A favorite dildo (called a "consolateur") is a hollowed glass tube filled with warm water!

Some women go for erotic balls (or hard-boiled hen's eggs) which they insert in their vaginas. Then they swing in a swing (or rock themselves vigorously in a rocking chair), vibrating themselves to a state of high excitement. Pigeon's eggs are called "pommes d'amour" (apples of love).

Clitoral masturbators go for tickling and titillation that involves rubbing the clitoris (that tiny female penis, as it's been called) with finger or some other instrument. They like sitting on a heel. Or rubbing their legs and thighs together. Or other body torsion -- on the corner of a chair, say, or against a piece of furniture. Or against a key in the bureau drawer, a knot in the chemise, hobby horse, swing, seesaw, Alma public school desk, etc. Even a tight lacing of corsets can suffice (it conjests the whole pelvic region).

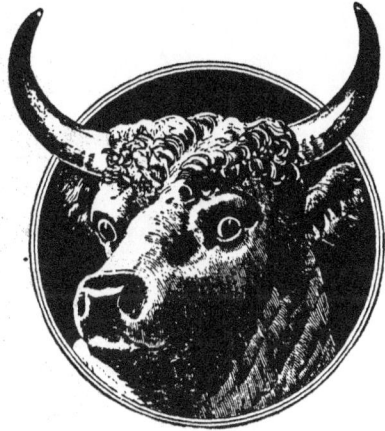

Urethral masturbation (sexual stimulation of the urethra, the tube that runs from the bladder to the surface of the body) is less frequently discussed, but obviously long popular. In 1862, a German surgeon invented a special instrument designed to extract hair pins from female bladders! One of the dangers of urethral masturbation (WARNING!!!) is that the urethra tends to "swallow" small objects -- hairpins, toothpicks, bodkins, etc. -- at the moment of orgasm.

But an imaginative woman can find orgasm nearly anywhere. Prolonged dancing or riding can set a woman off -- riding horses (real or hobby), trains, buses, automobiles. Or bikes, especially if the seat is high and tilted to contact the clitoris. Or climbing a pole. Or listening to music. Or thinking sexual thoughts. Or writing articles about masturbation. Or rocking (including rocking infants, which gives a new perspective on the popularity of the Madonna and Child image!).

Sitting or remaining in bed a long time can stir desire as can working on a sewing machine -- especially those old pedal machines! Witness this: Part of a superintendent's duty in a French sewing factory was to make the working women sit properly. If he failed, suddenly a machine would be heard going at a great velocity. It's pedaler would have that glazed, convulsive look in her eye. Her face would grow pale, and suddenly, she'd thrust her legs and hands out, give a suffocated cry and a long sigh that was usually little heard in the noise of the sewing room. So frequent was this occurrence, writes Havelock Ellis, that it was barely noticed.

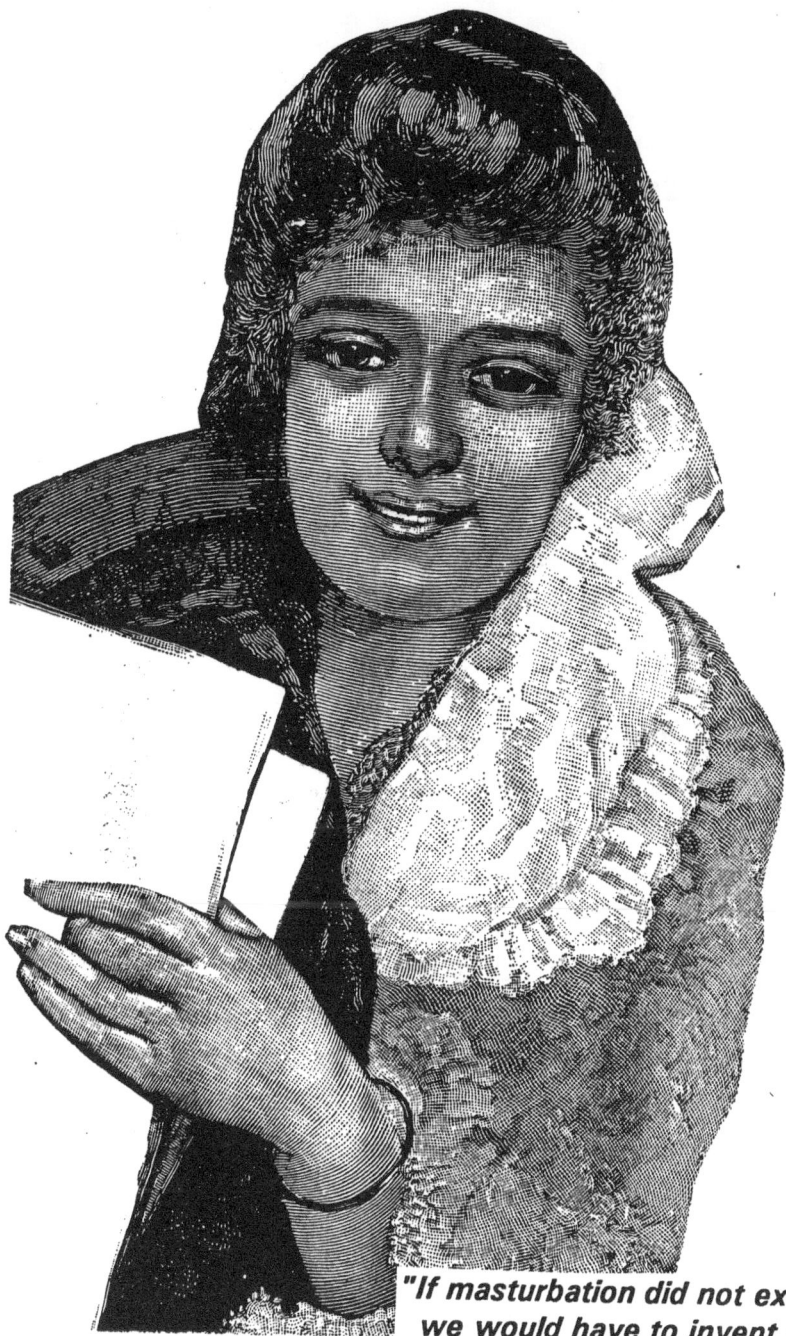

*"If masturbation did not exist,
we would have to invent it."*

from *Sexual Self-Stimulation*
edited by R. E. L. Masters

WARNING:

Not to be Read by Churches

This is a true story:

Went to print a post card
a post card of my poem
called "Masturbation Poem."

It reads:

"A clit in hand
is worth 2 in bush."

A cheery poem.

The sort of thing
that might brighten
a person's day
if she got it in the mail.

But I was afraid.

Would the postman
deliver it?

I mean,
is this a dirty poem
or what?
in the U. S. of A.

Nearly threw my idea
out.

But it nagged me.

Could I or couldn't I
mail a masturbation card?

I mean, legally.

Called up the Post Office
the Omaha branch
asked for information.

"Yes?" he said.

"I want to print a post card
but I need to know
what's legal
to send through the mail."

"Anything's legal but
Dirty Words," he said.

"Yes, but what's dirty?
I mean, is the word
M A S T U R B A T I O N
dirty?"

"Nah," he said.
"Masturbation,
that's a medical term,
isn't it?"

"Yes," I said,
quite willing
(under the circumstances)
to agree,

"but what about clit?"

"Clit?"

I spelled it.

"C-L-I-T.
Short for clitoris."

"Well, I don't know
off hand
about that."

"And bush?"

"Bush? Bush's
not dirty."

"But in the poem
bush has a sexual
connotation."

"I see. . . .
I think I better
speak to my supervisor."

"Maybe you'd like to hear
the poem first.
It's short."

"Okay," he said.

I read it to him.

"Masturbation Poem

"A clit in hand
is worth 2 in bush."

"Hold, please."

After a considerable while,
the post office official
returned.

"It's okay," he said.
"You can send it through the mail --
as long as you don't send any
to churches."

"Churches?"

"Yah, or anybody else
that might get offended
and make a complaint.
As long as no one complains,
it's okay."

"I see."

Then we spoke in unison:

"It's just a saying, anyway." (He)

"The poet's name will be
on the card." (Me)

A double moment
of shocked silence
as each heard the other.

Then he spoke:

"You mean someone WROTE that?"

"Yes," I admitted,
a bit shy, a bit proud,
wondering if he'd retract
his permission.

But he didn't,
so I printed
my Masturbation Card.

Only a quarter each,
five for a buck --

but you must promise
not to send any to churches!

Masturbation Poem

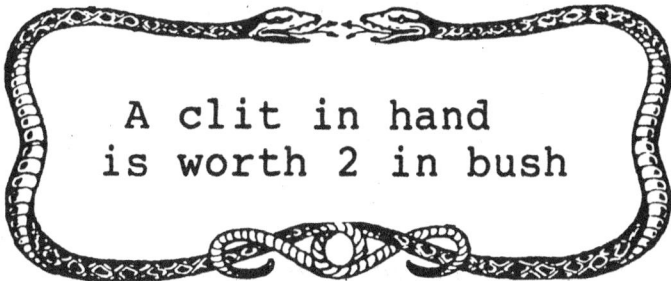

A clit in hand
is worth 2 in bush

Marilyn Coffey is author of the novel, *Marcella*, the first novel in the history of English literature to deal with female masturbation as part of the work's main theme. This ground-breaking book also deals with the theme of sexual abuse (by the minister).

Coffey also writes nonfiction and poetry. *Her Great Plain Patchwork: A Memoir* appeared from Iowa State University Press in 1989. *A Cretan Cycle: Fragments Unearthed from Knossos*, a book-length poem, was published by Bandanna Books of California in 1991. *Mail-Order Kid*, her biography of a Orphan Train Rider, appeared in 2010.